Pain Relief
Pain Management

Brian Birchmeier, CHt

DEDICATION

To my family. My constant inspiration and purpose.

CONTENTS

ACKNOWLEDGMENTS

My clients are a constant source of information, feedback and inspiration to fill the void of knowledge that is me – Thank you for that.

1 OPENING CREDITS

Opening Credits:

Welcome to the Maximum Performance Hypnotherapy Program: Pain Management, Written and Narrated by Brian Birchmeier.

To the casual reader who may have purchased this book for either self use or as a practitioner interested in providing Pain Relief and Pain Management techniques to your clients I must lead in with the caveat that this information in book form is required in order to publish audio books for Audible and that is the purpose for writing in this manner.

If you can use these words to improve your life or the lives of those around you then I applaud you and am grateful to be included.

The format for the rest of this book is as a series of scripts that we used in producing the audio book and we've included some bonus scripts because Createspace requires a specific number of pages in order to publish.

Be well!

Brian Birchmeier

2 INTRODUCTION

Welcome to the Pain Management session from Maximum Performance Hypnotherapy.

Pain Management has been a growing part of my practice, particularly from within my own family – and perhaps more to the point – from family members who don't believe in the hocus pocus, as they call it, of hypnotherapy.

My son is a scientist in Kinesiology and very much an empiricist – if you can't quantify it in peer reviewed literature – it didn't happen. The idea of anecdotal results absolutely mystifies him.

He and I have both been involved in Powerlifting and weight training for many years and during a session he injured his back, froze right up between his shoulder blades and was obviously in extreme pain. Unable to relieve the pain himself and fearing a trip to the hospital he allowed me to guide him into a light state of hypnosis as he laid painfully on the floor, provide the same instructions as you will receive here, and his words as he returned to outer awareness were: "I don't know why I don't hurt".

I'm not going to say "I told you so" here either – I promise.

Recently my father, who at 83 years of age considers anyone who can be hypnotized to be weak willed, had surgery to reduce impingements of nerves at three of the lumbar vertebral joints. He was reco9vering well but due to allergies that he had to many of the traditional pain medications he was miserable, unable to sleep and in general – a joy to be around. Finally the pain became strong enough that when I offered assistance his only statement was a gruff: "Come On".

He lay in bed and within just a few minutes he returned to outer awareness, looking very relaxed and with a bright smile he said: "No more pain, now let me get some sleep". He didn't take so much as an aspirin through the rest of his recovery and as you'll learn here, wherever and whenever he has pain such as headaches or arthritis flare ups he simply follows the steps himself and faster than a pain pill the pain is diminished if not gone altogether.

My wife recently learned that she has a form of liver disease which thankfully can be managed through diet and exercise but she really shouldn't take pain relievers. For a few weeks she diligently pushed through the pain in her hips and knees but it was becoming frustrating. As with the others she arrived at the point in which she was in enough pain to accept a hypnosis session. She experienced relief like the others and I think that you'll see that it makes sense as to why as I explain the process.

Pain Management is a short process; you do not need to be very deep into hypnosis to affect the pain receptors in your brain. The induction will be very short, just a few minutes of visualization and then instructions to your subconscious and you'll enjoy relieve immediately.

Let's talk for a moment about how any kind of anesthesia or analgesia works. This is not intended to be a scientific dissertation but I believe that this simple explanation will make sense.

Remember the question from your introduction to philosophy class first proposed as a thought experiment by Philosopher George Berkeley, in his work, *A Treatise Concerning the Principles of Human Knowledge* way back in(1710). If a tree falls in the forest and there is no one there to hear it – does it make a sound?

Far from the resounding 'duh' that I usually get when I repeat this question – that answer is quite instructive.

Sound, you see, only exists in your mind. Until your mind interprets the vibrations as you perceive it – the things that impact your tympanic membrane and its various ally's to facilitating your hearing – they are just that – vibrations. The vibrations exist but the sound does not until there is a device of some sort – such as your ear and the brain it serves, to convert & interpret the vibrations as sound.

If the question were changed to ask: It a tree falls in the forest and there is no one there, does it make vibrations the answer would be a resounding 'Yes'; All due respect given to Schrodinger's cat and the assorted quantum physicists who may be listening.

The idea of turning of pain is exactly the same concept. Employing chemical anesthesia, a general anesthetic that you would receive for a major surgery like my Dad's or a local given by your dentist before a procedure both do essentially the same thing – they interrupt the pain signals being sent by the injured part of your body. They don't allow the brain to interpret the signals as pain.

The signals are being sent – your jaw doesn't hold a conference and say: 'fellows let's just withhold sending the pain signals following that shot, it's obvious this chap has no interest in our situation'. Not a bit of it. The offended nerves are throwing out signals at a tremendous pace – there is simply no one answering the phone in the brain.

Hypnosis acts the same way. It simply instructs the brain to not react to the pain signals it is being sent.

You may use this technique for a headache – it works wonderfully even for migraines. You may use it post surgical or even for dental work – although I strongly encourage you speak with your dentist before scheduling the appointment. Many are fine with it – several are not.

You'll notice as you enjoy this session that I'll say: If it is important that you feel some pain so that you do not further injure yourself, then do, but limit the pain to only the smallest amount.

This instruction is here for two reasons, the obvious 1st reason is that pain exists for a reason and to remove it totally is simply irresponsible. The 2nd reason is that athletes will sometimes attempt to use these techniques to "get back in the game" and risk further injury – don't do it.

That brings me to the important disclaimer that this session is not intended to replace, diagnose or treat medical conditions or illness. If you have medical questions please contact your physician.

And finally, before we begin the session, allow me to describe what you'll experience, particularly for those who've not enjoyed hypnotherapy before.

Hypnosis looks on the outside as if someone is sleeping, but that is about as far as the similarities go. You'll still be fully aware of your surroundings, you'll hear outside noises and your conscious mind will still be worrying about what you have to do after you listen to this just as it has been while you've endured this introduction. That will be particularly true in this session as we will not be going deeply into hypnosis.

The session will, however, begin to open, what I call, an inner awareness that makes much of the activity of the conscious mind, well, let's just say – not quite as important.

I hope that you'll enjoy this program and share it with whomever you feel may benefit from it – although please don't copy it without permission as it is covered by copyright protections 2017.

As you find relief please go back to the site from which you purchased this program and give it a review – your feedback is valuable and particularly in this case – could make the difference between someone suffering needlessly with pain that could otherwise have been relieved.

Take some time as well to browse the Audible bookstore and iTunes for other programs from Maximum Performance Hypnotherapy – particularly our popular 4x4 series.

With that it's about time to begin. We'll record the actual session as a separate chapter so that when you listen again it will be easy to locate.

This should be obvious but absolutely no listening to this session while driving or operating machinery of any kind. It is very powerful.

3 PAIN RELIEF / PAIN MANAGEMENT – THE SESSION

Pain Management Hypnotherapy Session

Find a comfortable position. One that allows you to relax and be comfortable and as you settle in I'd like to bring your attention to your breathing.

Notice your breathing in and out.

As you focus on your breathing and you settle in for your session note that from time to time you may feel a wiggle of have to move and if that occurs feel free to move, hypnosis is not a state of being immobile.

As you focus on your breathing notice that you are breathing in relaxation and breathing out tension...

Breathing in relaxation through your nose and breathing our tension through your mouth

In through your nose

Out through your mouth

Deeper and deeper

More and more relaxed

Every cycle of breathing takes you much deeper – twice as deep as you were before

You continue to listen to the sound of my voice and you feel very relaxed, very comfortable

As you continue to go deeper and deeper I'd like for you to visualize for me that you are at the top of a stairwell, each cycle of breathing taking you deeper and deeper

As you observe your surroundings, looking around with your mind's eye, look up and notice construction of the ceiling – it may be tiled or painted, it may be wood or open sky. Take a moment to observe the ceiling, all the while going deeper and deeper, more and more relaxed.

Look down now and notice your feet – you may be wearing shoes – or perhaps you have bare feet.

See yourself standing at the top of the stairwell, looking down at your feet and get a sense of being grounded as you stand there. Deeper and deeper, more and more relaxed

Notice the construction of the stairs. They may wooden or steel, concrete? They may be painted or carpeted.

Notice the walls – they may be painted or wall papered. Notice the texture, deeper and deeper, more and more relaxed.

As you continue to relax bring your attention back to your breath for a moment – continuing to breathe in relaxation and out tension.

And notice, off in the distance a doorway. Each time you breathe in you not only go deeper but you bring the doorway closer

And each time you breathe out you are more and more relaxed and the doorway opens slightly more.

In a moment we will walk down the steps and with each step you be twice as deep twice as relaxed and the doorway will be closer and closer and will be open more and more.

By the time we reach the bottom of the stairs the doorway will be very close and on the other side you'll see a wonderful safe place, one in which your conscious mind will feel very comfortable and when we arrive just allow your conscious mind to go into that wonderful safe place and it can do all of the things it needs to do. Sometimes it will pay attention to the sound of my voice and sometimes not – either way is fine, your subconscious will be doing all of the work.

You may hear noises from outside of this recording or even from your own mind during this session and that is perfectly normal, just stay focused on the sound of my voice and let those noises just be in the background and allow them to take you deeper and deeper as you do with each breath and with each word that you hear from me.

Lets get started and go from step 10 to step 9 – deeper and deeper

Step 9 to step 8 – more and more relaxed

Step 7 see the doorway being closer

Step 6 the doorway opens a bit more each time

5 breathing in relaxation

4 breathing our tension

3 deeper and deeper

2 more and more relaxed and

1 and allow your conscious mind to go into that wonderful safe place.

As you continue to relax I'd like for you to bring your attention back to your breath

Notice how your breath feels as you breathe in – notice where you feel it – your nose, your mouth, your chest your lungs

30

Now I would like for you to bring your attention to your dominant hand – if you right handed then your right hand. Left handed then your left.

Focus your attention on your hand and in a few moments you'll notice that it feels a bit different. It may be a tingle, it may feel as if there is a glove over your hand – but in moment you'll experience the hand feeling different from the other.

I'll give you a few moments just to be with that sensation

60

As you continue to have your dominant hand be the object of your awareness imagine that the hand has a glove over it and when it feels this way – any part of your body that the hand and glove touch or cover will immediately enjoy relief from any pain.

Now if you can physically reach and touch the part of you that is experiencing pain – do so. If you can't reach it just imagine that your hand moves to the affected area and it will have the exact same affect.

If there is an injury or if there is something that your doctor should observe – leave just enough pain so that the affected body part reminds you of the situation and that you get the proper care as soon as possible. Leave only enough pain to get your attention – otherwise remove it.

And now relax, the pain is gone or greatly diminished.

If you find that you need to employ pain management again simply find a safe and quiet place where you can relax for a few moments. Close your eyes and take a few deep healing relaxing breaths and when you do – notice that sensation in your dominant hand. Notice that feeling and once you are aware of that feeling then move the hand either literally or in your mind over the part of your body that requires relief and the pain is simply turned off.

The next time you listen to one of these recordings and it is safe to go into a very deep state of hypnosis and you hear me say the words MPH sleep now you will instantly drop deeper into a state of hypnosis than you have ever been before.

In just a few moments I will count from 1 to 5 and when I reach 5 you'll open your eyes feeling wonderfully relaxed, pain free and energetic. If it is time to go to sleep you'll find yourself easily and effortlessly falling into a deep healing restful sleep.

And now its time to return to outer awareness, I'll count from 1 to 5 and when I reach 5 you'll open your eyes and feel wonderful, pain free and energetic.

1 you are free from pain

2 you are in control of all of your perceptions

3 you are happy and energetic

4 smile you are almost there and

5 – open your eyes feeling wonderful in every way.

4 CLOSING CREDITS

Closing Credits: Thank you for listening; this has been the Maximum Performance Hypnotherapy Program: Pain Management. Written and Narrated by Brian Birchmeier, Copyright 2017, Performance Copyright 2017 by Maximum Performance Hypnotherapy.

5 BONUS SCRIPT: BUSINESS SUCCESS

Bonus Script: Business Success

As you listen to the sound of my voice you will continue to go deeper and deeper into that wonderful state of therapeutic hypnosis where wonderful changes take place easily and effortlessly to improve the areas of your life that are important to you.

And as you relax you realize that all of the learning experiences that you've experienced in your life are necessary for you to be at this place in time. You have accepted all of the learning experiences that were unpleasant, understanding that without those experiences you could not enjoy the success that you create. Business Success is a directly related to the problems that you are able to solve and you understand that without problems there is no business.

Your ability to consistently and effectively create systems and processes to successfully fulfill the needs and desires of more and more people consistently provides wonderful rewards. The rewards of satisfaction and humility – knowing that because of you the lives of many people are better. The lives of your customers and clients, the lives of your employees, the lives that are impacted as a result of the benefits you've created for your customers, clients and employees.

You understand that money is a motivational tool when money was tight – particularly at the beginning. As your business grows and your financial needs are satisfied wonderful other incentives to continue your success have developed that are even more compelling than money ever had been. Take a few moments and give thought to all of the important things that motivate you beyond having your basic needs met.

Your position as a role model to others; Your family, your friends, your children, your employees, your community all benefit from the example that you set.

Your position today provides the perfect place to develop your successes of tomorrow.

You have developed a foundation of HONESTY in all of your business practices. You are tremendously disciplined in your assessment of all of your business interests. You insist on accurate and effective accounting that always allows you to know the status of your enterprise. When you see other business owners deceiving themselves or others by not recognizing the true state of their business it reinforces your resolve to be true to yourself, your family, your business, your community in all circumstances. Only with true representations of your business can you ever hope to build a truly successful and sustained business.

Your clarity of the Mission, Vision, Values and Culture of your organization is crystal clear. Your clarity is apparent in all that you do and it resonates through your entire organization. This clarity from the most entry level person to the very top of your organization makes priorities very clear and evident, and distractions are dismissed before they ever adversely affect the business.

Your clarity of Mission, Vision, Values and Culture make building your team a pleasure and in instances where mistakes are made in building that team, they are quickly identified and eliminated – the mistakes cannot prevail in an environment of strong Mission, Vision, Values and

Culture.

Your clarity makes the constant Research and Development of new products and services, systems and processes and the ability to discern the results of R&D that are congruent with your current practices and Mission, Vision, Values and Culture and those that can be sold or deployed elsewhere for royalties and revenue, and those that need to be discarded; all of these decisions are very clear, very concise, very accurate and very powerful.

Your clarity makes the evaluation on ongoing products and services, systems and processes, effective. You are able to discern easily and effortlessly the parts of your business that are no longer in the best interests of the enterprise and you are able to effectively and efficiently terminate them.

Your clarity of purpose makes the gathering of information, market data and demographics enjoyable and effective along with the wisdom to ensure that the Purpose, Mission, Vision, Values and Culture of your organization and strengthened with each decision made.

Your commitment to your Purpose, Mission, Vision, Values and Culture prevents hubris from ever taking hold in the organization. You have been wise to implement the systems and processes to deal with any instance that you or your team identifies evidence of any negative or non-congruent or non-business enhancing energy or element in your organization.

Your gift of humility makes you comfortable in the knowledge that your success is dependent upon all of the other people involved in the process – from customers to your team and partners & advisors. Your humility perfectly balances the appropriate pride of accomplishment and completely eliminates any hubris that may develop.

Your success is assured.

6 BONUS SCRIPT: FEARLESS SALES

Bonus Script: Fearless Sales

Ego Strengthening: You are now so VERY DEEPLY ASLEEP....that EVERYTHING that I tell you.... That is going to happen to you....FOR YOUR OWN GOOD.....WILL happen...EXACTLY as I tell you. And EVERY FEELING ...that I tell you that you will experience....you WILL experience EXACTLY as I tell you. And these same things WILL CONTINUE TO HAPPEN TO YOU....EVERY DAY...and you WILL CONTINUE TO EXPERIENCE these same feelings...EVERY DAY....JUST AS STRONGLY...JUST as surely...JUST as powerfully...when you are at home, or at work....as when you are with me in this room.

Fear of rejection is a natural part of life. In early human history being rejected by our peers often meant starvation, exposure to predators and death. We are hardwired to survive and that is why as you understand the origins of the fear, any aspect of that fear appearing instantly triggers your confidence. Instantly and effortlessly triggers your Charisma. Instantly and effortlessly brings the exact body language to bear, the perfect words to your lips and instantly and effortlessly brings calm, confidence and the ability to do the things that your success requires.

You have developed an exceptional; WORLD CLASS ability and this

WORL CLASS ABILITY allows and requires you to be absolutely FEARLESS in Sales Situations. You take control easily and effortlessly and yet appear so comfortable, so relaxed so at ease and the people you are dealing with instantly like and trust you. You make it look so easy – even though you have worked hard at your craft for many years, countless hours of practice, critique, improvement and success.

Your Preparation is exceptional allowing you to make sure that the focus of the communication is always on your prospect, ensuring that they feel important, happy, heard, safe and secure.

You are an expert in your field. Knowledge of your offerings is your competitive advantage you take every opportunity to increase your skills, knowledge and implementation of all that you have to offer your customers and clients.

Your expertise is valuable and you enjoy the fruits of your labors, skills and dedication. You earn vast amounts of revenue and you continually earn large incomes as you provide far more value through your knowledge, skills and offerings.

You see others in your profession who satisfy themselves with just being OK, or just getting by and being aware of their complacency shields you from your own. You provide expert knowledge, skills and world class offerings and you enjoy the fruits of your high standards. Shakespeare said "To Thine Own Self Be True, and then it must follow, the night the day though canst not be false to any man". You are true to yourself – honest with yourself and with everyone that you contact – thanks just good business, and when others say "good enough", you persist. You are being true to yourself. When others meet their quotas and goals early and quit – you persist knowing that they are only hurting themselves. You are being true to yourself.

You are the role model that others choose to follow.

Your body language reinforces all that you do and say. Your mind instantly connects and interprets the needs and concerns of the people with whom you are in contact and your body language expresses that perfectly.

Your confidence radiates from every aspect of your being. The people with whom you come into contact feel like the most important people in the world, and you know that the more important they feel about themselves when they are with you, the more important you are to them and the more important you are to them the more likely they are to do good business with you.

Any doubt that enters your mind immediately makes you stronger, more confident, more charismatic and better prepared, instantly annihilating any doubt. Ant this takes place instantly and subconsciously so that your conscious mind does not need to bother and you may never know that it takes place, but your inner confidence assures Fearlessness in Sales is effortless and instantaneous – it is the natural and real you.

7 MPH GENERAL INDUCTION

For Hypnotherapy Professionals – the Maximum Performance Hypnotherapy General Induction:

Hello and welcome to Maximum Performance Hypnotherapy.

We are happy to provide these recordings for your use free of charge and we encourage you to share these with anyone that may benefit from them. We encourage you to email any suggestions for programs that would be beneficial to you to results@maxphy.com or to use the "Contact Us" page of our website at www.maxphy.com.

It is very important that you listen to these recordings only when safe to do so and NEVER when operating any type of machinery or vehicle.

These recordings are very powerful and you can expect spectacular results. If, however, you find a part of you resisting the change or feel yourself slow or cease to make progress, contact us immediately for a personal Hypnotherapeutic Session to remove the roadblocks. Reach out to us for help. For optimal results listen to this recording for at least 21 days to ensure the results that are important to you.

This material is copyrighted 2015, Maximum Performance Hypnotherapy, LLC.

And now, if you are in a safe environment, it is time for you to begin your journey toward creating the changes that are so important to you.

Make yourself comfortable and begin to concentrate on your breathing. Your eyes will begin to relax and close on their own – just allow it to happen. Feel the wonderful relaxation flowing into you as you breathe in and all tension leaving your body as you breathe out.

Breathe in through your nose, out through your mouth. You are breathing easily and effortlessly, more and more comfortably. Allow your body to move as it needs to. You will remain perfectly balanced throughout this process and your body will be a perfect temperature for you – not too hot, not too cold. You are perfectly relaxed and perfectly comfortable.

MPH Sleep Now – go into a very deep state of relaxation, deeper than you've ever been before, go into the deepest state of therapeutic hypnosis that exists so that you may quickly and easily bring about the changes that are important to you.

You may feel a wonderful wave of relaxation just above your forehead and as it moves down over you, relaxing everything quickly and easily, feel the relaxation of your forehead – all the muscles just relax and feel the relaxation throughout your whole head, relaxing your scalp flowing over your cheeks – relaxing all of the muscles around your eyes, relaxing your jaw – all of the tension stored in your jaws just melts away, your jaw may fall open and that's ok. You'll breathe, swallow and relax perfectly without having to think about any of it.

Feel the relaxation flowing over your neck and across your shoulders, releasing all of the tension in your neck and shoulders – it all just melts away. You are at peace. You are safe and secure moving quickly and easily into that therapeutic realm of hypnosis where wonderful changes take place easily and effortlessly.

The relaxation is flowing down your upper arms, forearms and relaxing all of those muscles in your hands. You are warm and comfortable, perfectly balanced, safe and at peace.

The relaxation is flowing over your chest and abdomen – relaxing all of the muscles and every part of your body, front to back, side to side. The large muscles of your back completely relax releasing any tension or pain, perfectly supporting all of your body's structures while allowing you to relax deeper and deeper into that wonderful therapeutic realm of hypnosis.

Feel the relaxation flowing over your hips, your thighs; relaxing all of the muscles in your hips and legs, just melting and feeling wonderful.

Feel the relaxation flowing over your lower legs and into your feet as if you were getting a wonderful foot massage, relaxing all of the muscles in your feet and legs, melting, warm and comfortably into that wonderful state of relaxation and hypnosis where changes happen.

And now I'd like for you to focus on a spot on your forehead, just above the bridge of your nose – focus your eyes on that spot as you listen to the sound of my voice. All of the other sounds around you simply help you to relax even more – they aren't important. Your conscious mind may not even be listening all of the time and that's ok, your subconscious mind hears everything and will be working to bring about the changes that are important to you.

As you focus on that spot on your forehead your eyes will begin to get tired, fatigued – that's ok, just stay focused for as long as you can. As you stay focused you'll feel the muscles around your eyes just relax, relax to the point where it just feels great to leave your eyes closed, and while you know that you could open them at any time – it's just too much work.

And now, notice that there is a beautiful light above your head, allow your subconscious to choose whatever color that light should be to bring about the changes that are important to you, it could be many colors – and the colors can change at any time to help facilitate the process.

And imagine that your body is like a mist in the morning and the light is

27

like the sun shining through that mist and as the light shines through the mist that is you, it instantly relaxes every molecule, from front to back, side to side, all at once as time just ceases to be important.

See the light shining on your forehead, relaxing all of the muscles of your forehead and scalp, front and back as the mist that is you receive the light all at the same time.

The light moves behind your eyes, relaxing your mind and your body, relaxing all of the muscles of your face, around your eyes, your jaws – releasing any remaining tension in your jaws. The light moves down your neck and shoulders instantly releasing any tension remaining there and in your back.

Feel the light moving down your upper arms, then your forearms moving into your hands and shooting right out of your fingertips. See the light beginning to form a protective sphere around you – protecting you and enabling you to bring about the changes that are important to you.

The light moves down your chest and abdomen relaxing the entire core of your body, relaxing your back and centering in mid abdomen – your solar plexus. Protecting you, guiding you and bringing about the changes that are important to you.

The light moves down across your hips relaxing all of the muscles of your hips and upper legs, the light moves through the mist that are your legs and travels through your lower legs, into your feet, relaxing all of the muscles in your feet and shooting right out of your toes, adding to the light from your fingers and solar plexus completing a wonderful sphere of light that will allow anything unpleasant, unproductive or harmful to leave without hindrance, but protecting all that is helpful, beneficial and life enhancing – allowing only good to be there and facilitating the changes that are important to you.

I would ask that any of your spiritual guides, guardian angels, teachers, masters, friends or relatives who may assist in this process, be present to protect you and to facilitate the changes that are important you, according to your personal belief system.

ABOUT THE AUTHOR

I am is first and foremost a husband and a father. I'm apparently unendingly curious and truly enjoy the life of being a serial entrepreneur.

My wife Bonnie and I celebrated our 30th anniversary this year and our greatest pleasure and success is in our children, all three grown and out of the home, doing well and exploring their own paths.

We live on a small farm that we are in the process of converting from hay to hardwoods and by about the year 2067 it should be quite impressive.

My Hypnotherapy practice is an enjoyable segment of my business interests, in fact I think it is safe to say that I run that part of my life as a vocation rather than a business. I also publish magazines for a living and enjoy consulting for small businesses; those with sales of up to $10 million per year.

I've retired from Powerlifting Competitions, although it isn't unusual for me to start training periodically – there is always one more tournament, one more record to break isn't there?

My passion as a hobby for the last several years has been General Aviation and as a pilot and proud owner of a 1965 Cessna 150, you are as likely to find me in the air in my free time as anywhere.

If we happen to run into each other, please say 'Hi' – in the mean time:

Be well!

Brian Birchmeier

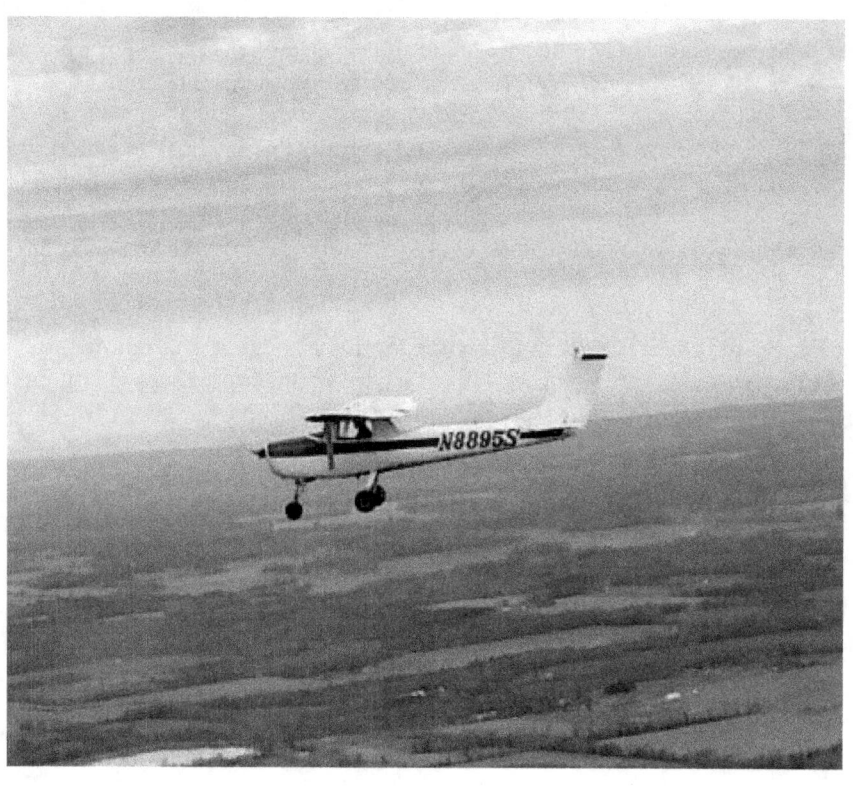

www.ingramcontent.com/pod-product-compliance
Lightning Source LLC
Chambersburg PA
CBHW061928280526
45787CB00004B/1529